INSTANT

FLAT BELLY

RECIPES

10 Flat Belly Foods To Incorporate Into Your Diet For A Trimmer Waistline

Dr. Judith Elvis

DISCLAIMER

CONTENT

Instant Flat Belly Recipes

Introduction

Are you looking to slim down your waistline and get an instant flat belly? Achieving a flat belly can be challenging, but incorporating certain foods into your diet can make it easier to achieve your goal. In this article, we will introduce to you instant flat belly foods that can help you get a trimmer waistline. These flat-belly foods can help you slim down your waistline by providing essential nutrients and helping you feel satisfied and full. Many of these foods are high in fiber, which can help regulate digestion and keep you feeling full for longer periods. They are also rich in nutrients like antioxidants, healthy fats, and protein, which can help support weight loss and overall health. By incorporating these flat-belly foods into your diet, you can take an important step toward achieving your health and wellness goals. So, without further ado, let's get started on discovering these instant flat belly foods!

Chapter 1
Leafy Greens

Leafy greens like spinach, kale, and broccoli are some of the best flat-belly foods you can include in your diet. These nutrient-rich vegetables are low in calories and high in fiber, making them a great choice for weight loss and a flat belly. In addition to helping you feel full and satisfied, leafy greens are packed with antioxidants and other nutrients that can support overall health. They are also a great source of vitamin K, which can help keep bones strong and healthy. Try adding a handful of leafy greens to your smoothies, salads, or roasted vegetables for an easy and tasty way to boost your intake of these flat-belly foods.

There are so many types of leafy greens to choose from, so you won't get bored easily. Some other options to consider include:

- Arugula
- Collard greens
- Romaine lettuce
- Swiss chard
- Mustard greens
- Watercress

Leafy greens are also extremely versatile and can be used in a variety of dishes. Try using them as a base for salads, adding them to sandwiches or wraps, or sautéing them with garlic and olive oil as a side dish. You can even incorporate leafy greens into your breakfast by adding them to omelets or smoothie bowls. The options are endless, so don't be afraid to get creative and try new ways to

incorporate leafy greens into your meals

Chapter 2
Berries

Berries are another excellent choice for flat-belly foods. These sweet and delicious fruits are packed with fiber, which can help keep you feeling full and satisfied. They are also rich in antioxidants, which can help protect your body from damaging free radicals. Some of the best berries for a flat belly include strawberries, raspberries, and blackberries. These types of berries are lower in sugar compared to some other options, making them a better choice for weight loss and a flat belly.

In addition to their fiber and antioxidant content, berries are also a great source of vitamin C, which can help support a healthy immune system and promote healthy skin. Try adding a handful of berries to your oatmeal, smoothies, or yogurt for a tasty and nutritious boost. You can also eat them on their own as a tasty and healthy snack.

Other types of berries that can be included in a flat belly diet include:

- Blueberries
- Cranberries
- Goji berries
- Acai berries

Like leafy greens, berries are extremely versatile and can be used in a variety of dishes. You can add them to your breakfast cereal or oats, blend them into smoothies or smoothie bowls, or use them as a topping for yogurt or oatmeal. You can also incorporate berries into your baking, such as making muffins or adding them to pancakes. They can also be a delicious addition to salads or as a topping for grilled chicken or fish. The possibilities are endless, so don't be afraid to get creative and try new ways to include berries in your meals.

Chapter 3

Avocados

Avocados are another excellent choice for flat-belly foods. These creamy and delicious fruits are high in healthy fats, which can help keep you feeling full and satisfied. They are also a good source of fiber, which can aid in digestion and support weight loss. In addition to their flat-belly benefits, avocados are also a great source of potassium, which can help regulate blood pressure and support heart health.

One of the great things about avocados is that they are extremely versatile and can be used in a variety of dishes. You can mash them up and use them as a spread on toast or sandwiches, add them to salads or bowls, or use them as a topping for tacos or burritos. You can even blend them into smoothies or make homemade guacamole. Just be mindful of the serving size, as avocados are high in calories and fat. Aim to include a small amount of avocado in your meals rather than overindulging.

Another way to incorporate avocados into your diet is by using them as a substitute for other less healthy ingredients. For example, you can use mashed avocado as a replacement for mayonnaise in sandwiches or as a base for homemade dips. You can also use avocado as a replacement for butter in baking recipes, as it can add a creamy and rich texture to cookies and brownies. Just be sure to adjust the amount you use, as avocados may have a stronger flavor than the ingredient you are replacing.

Overall, avocados are a tasty and nutritious addition to a flat-belly diet. Just be sure to watch your portion sizes and include them in moderation as part of a well-rounded and balanced diet.

Chapter 4

Nuts and Seeds

Nuts and seeds are another excellent choice for flat belly foods. These small but mighty snacks are packed with fiber, protein, and healthy fats, which can help keep you feeling full and satisfied. They are also a good source of nutrients like magnesium, potassium, and iron, which can support overall health. Some of the best nuts and seeds for a flat belly include almonds, chia seeds, and flax seeds.

Nuts and seeds can be a convenient and tasty snack option when you're on the go. Just be mindful of portion sizes, as they are high in calories and fat. A serving size of nuts and seeds is generally about 1-2 ounces, or a small handful.

You can also incorporate nuts and seeds into your meals by adding them to salads, oatmeal, yogurt, or smoothies. They can also be used as a topping for roasted vegetables or baked goods, or as a base for homemade energy bars. Just be sure to choose unsalted options to control your sodium intake.

Other types of nuts and seeds that can be included in a flat belly diet include:

- Walnuts
- Pistachios
- Cashews
- Sunflower seeds
- Pumpkin seeds

Like other flat belly foods, nuts and seeds are extremely versatile and can be used in a variety of dishes. You can add them to your breakfast cereal or oats, blend them into smoothies or smoothie bowls, or use them as a topping for yogurt or oatmeal. You can also incorporate nuts and seeds into your baking, such as making muffins or adding them to pancakes. They can also be a delicious addition to salads or as a topping for grilled chicken or fish. The possibilities are endless, so don't be afraid to get creative and try new ways to include nuts and seeds in your meals. Just be sure to watch your portion sizes and include them in moderation as part of a well-rounded and balanced diet.

Chapter 5

Legumes

Legumes, such as beans, lentils, and chickpeas, are another excellent choice for flat belly foods. These plant-based protein sources are high in fiber, which can help keep you feeling full and satisfied. They are also a good source of nutrients like iron, potassium, and B vitamins, which can support overall health. Legumes are also low in calories and fat, making them a great choice for weight loss and a flat belly.

There are so many types of legumes to choose from, so you won't get bored easily. Some other options to consider include:

- Black beans

- Kidney beans

- Lima beans

- Peas

- Edamame

Legumes are extremely versatile and can be used in a variety of dishes. You can add them to soups, stews, and chili, or use them as a base for veggie burgers or falafel. You can also incorporate them into your meals by adding them to salads, bowls, or roasted vegetables. Also they can be mashed and used as a dip or spread. The options are endless, so don't be afraid to get creative and try new ways to include legumes in your meals. Just be sure to rinse and drain canned legumes to remove excess sodium.

Another way to incorporate legumes into your diet is by using them as a replacement for other less healthy ingredients. For example, you can use mashed legumes as a replacement for meat in dishes like tacos or pasta sauces. You can also use legumes as a replacement for other sources of protein in recipes, such as using chickpeas instead of chicken in a salad or using lentils instead of ground beef in a soup. Just be sure to adjust the amount you use, as legumes may have a different texture or flavor than the ingredient you are replacing.

Overall, legumes are a tasty and nutritious addition to a flat belly diet. They are a great source of plant-based protein and can help keep you feeling full and satisfied. Just be sure to include them as part of a well-rounded and balanced diet, and remember to rinse and drain canned legumes to remove excess sodium.

Chapter 6

Whole grains

Whole grains are another excellent choice for flat belly foods. These nutrient-rich grains are high in fiber, which can help keep you feeling full and satisfied. They are also a good source of nutrients like B vitamins, iron, and magnesium, which can support overall health. Some of the best whole grains for a flat belly include quinoa, oats, and brown rice.

Whole grains are extremely versatile and can be used in a variety of dishes. You can add them to soups and stews, use them as a base for bowls, or incorporate them into your baking. They can also be a delicious addition to salads or as a side dish with roasted vegetables or protein. Just be sure to choose whole grain options rather than refined grains, as whole grains are higher in nutrients and fiber and can be more beneficial for weight loss and a flat belly.

Incorporating whole grains into meal plan is easy. Just be sure to read labels carefully and choose options that list a whole grain as the first ingredient. You can also try experimenting with different types of whole grains to find ones you enjoy and to add variety to your meals.

Other types of whole grains that can be included in a flat belly diet include:

- Barley
- Buckwheat

- Bulgur

- Farro

- Millet

- Spelt

Like other flat belly foods, whole grains are extremely versatile and can be used in a variety of dishes. You can add them to your breakfast cereal or oats, blend them into smoothies or smoothie bowls, or use them as a topping for yogurt or oatmeal. You can also incorporate whole grains into your baking, such as making muffins or adding them to pancakes. They can also be a delicious addition to salads or as a side dish with grilled chicken or fish. The possibilities are endless, so don't be afraid to get creative and try new ways to include whole grains in your meals. Just be sure to choose whole grain options rather than refined grains, as whole grains are higher in nutrients and fiber and can be more beneficial for weight loss and a flat belly.

Chapter 7

Fermented Foods

Fermented foods, such as yogurt, kefir, and sauerkraut, are another excellent choice for flat belly foods. These foods are rich in probiotics, which are beneficial bacteria that can help support digestion and a healthy gut. A healthy gut can be important for weight loss and a flat belly, as it can help you absorb nutrients and feel satisfied and full. Fermented foods are also a good source of nutrients like calcium, protein, and vitamin D, which can support overall health.

Incorporating fermented foods into your meal plan is easy. You can try adding a serving of yogurt or kefir to your breakfast or using sauerkraut as a topping for sandwiches or bowls. You can also try incorporating other fermented foods into your meals, such as kimchi or pickles. Just be sure to choose options that are made with live and active cultures, as these will be the most beneficial for your gut health.

Overall, fermented foods are a tasty and nutritious addition to a flat belly diet. They are a great source of probiotics and can help support digestion and a healthy gut. Just be sure to choose options that are made with live and active cultures, and include fermented foods as part of a well-rounded and balanced diet.

Other types of fermented foods that can be included in a flat belly diet include:

- Kombucha

- Miso

- Tempeh

- Pickled vegetables

- Natto

Fermented foods are not only good for your gut health, but they can also add flavor and interest to your meals. You can use fermented foods as a condiment, such as adding miso to soups or using pickled vegetables as a topping for sandwiches. You can also try incorporating fermented foods into your cooking, such as using kombucha in marinades or using tempeh as a protein source in stir-fries. The possibilities are endless, so don't be afraid to get creative and try new ways to include fermented foods in your meals. Just be sure to choose options that are made with live and active cultures, and include fermented foods as part of a well-rounded and balanced diet.

Chapter 8

Healthy Fats

Including healthy fats in your diet can be important for weight loss and a flat belly. These fats, such as monounsaturated and polyunsaturated fats, can help keep you feeling full and satisfied and can also support overall health. Avocados, olive oil, nuts and seeds are the best sources of healthy fats.

Incorporating healthy fats into your diet is easy. You can try adding a serving of nuts or seeds to your meals or snacks or using olive oil as a dressing for salads or as a cooking oil. You can also try incorporating healthy fats into your meals by adding avocado to sandwiches or using it as a spread or topping. Just be mindful of portion sizes, as fats are high in calories and it's important to include them in moderation as part of a well-rounded and balanced diet.

Overall, healthy fats are an important part of a flat-belly diet. They can help keep you feeling full and satisfied and can also support overall health. Just be sure to choose healthy fat sources and include them in moderation as part of a well-rounded and balanced diet.

Other sources of healthy fats that can be included in a flat belly diet include:

- Olives
- Coconut oil

- Nut butter (such as peanut butter or almond butter)

- Flaxseed oil

- Sesame oil

Like other flat-belly foods, healthy fats are extremely versatile and can be used in a variety of dishes. You can add them to your breakfast cereal or oats, blend them into smoothies or smoothie bowls, or use them as a topping for yogurt or oatmeal. You can also incorporate healthy fats into your baking, such as using coconut oil as a replacement for butter in cookies or using nut butter as a filling for energy balls. They can also be a delicious addition to salads or as a topping for grilled chicken or fish. The possibilities are endless, so don't be afraid to get creative and try new ways to include healthy fats in your meals. Just be sure to choose healthy fat sources and

include them in moderation as part of a well-rounded and balanced diet.

Chapter 9

Lean Proteins

Including lean proteins in your diet can be important for weight loss and a flat belly. These proteins, such as chicken, turkey, and fish, are low in fat and calories and can help keep you feeling full and satisfied. They are also a good source of nutrients like iron, zinc, and B vitamins, which can support overall health.

Incorporating lean proteins into your diet is easy. You can try adding a serving of chicken, turkey, or fish to your meals or using them as a base for salads or bowls. You can also try incorporating other lean protein sources into your meals, such as tofu or eggs. Just be sure to choose protein sources that are low in fat and calories and

include them in moderation as part of a well-rounded and balanced diet.

Overall, lean proteins are an important part of a flat-belly diet. They can help keep you feeling full and satisfied and can also support overall health. Just be sure to choose lean protein sources and include them in moderation as part of a well-rounded and balanced diet.

Other sources of lean protein that can be included in a flat belly diet include:

- Tofu
- Beans and legumes
- Greek yogurt
- Cottage cheese

- Eggs

Like other flat-belly foods, lean proteins are extremely versatile and can be used in a variety of dishes. You can add them to your breakfast cereal or oats, blend them into smoothies or smoothie bowls, or use them as a topping for yogurt or oatmeal. You can also incorporate lean proteins into your baking, such as using tofu as a replacement for eggs in vegan recipes or using beans as a protein source in brownies. They can also be a delicious addition to salads or as a topping for roasted vegetables or grains. The possibilities are endless, so don't be afraid to get creative and try new ways to include lean proteins in your meals. Just be sure to choose lean protein sources and include them in moderation as part of a well-rounded and balanced diet.

Chapter 10
Spices and Seasonings

Including spices and seasonings in your diet can be important for weight loss and a flat belly. These flavorful ingredients can help add flavor to your meals without adding extra calories or fat. Some of the best spices and seasonings for a flat belly include cinnamon, turmeric, and ginger.

Incorporating spices and seasonings into your diet is easy. You can try adding a pinch of cinnamon to your oatmeal or smoothies, or using turmeric and ginger as a seasoning for roasted vegetables or stir-fries. You can also try incorporating other spices and seasonings into your meals, such as cumin, paprika, or garlic. Just be sure to choose spices and seasonings that are low in sodium and

include them in moderation as part of a well-rounded and balanced diet.

Overall, spices and seasonings are an important part of a flat belly diet. They can help add flavor to your meals without adding extra calories or fat and can also support overall health. Just be sure to choose low-sodium options and include them in moderation as part of a well-rounded and balanced diet.

Other types of spices and seasonings that can be included in a flat belly diet include:

- Cumin
- Paprika
- Garlic

- Chili powder

- Cardamom

- Coriander

Like other flat belly foods, spices and seasonings are extremely versatile and can be used in a variety of dishes. You can add them to your breakfast cereal or oats, blend them into smoothies or smoothie bowls, or use them as a topping for yogurt or oatmeal. You can also incorporate spices and seasonings into your baking, such as using cinnamon in cookies or adding paprika to roasted vegetables. They can also be a delicious addition to salads or as a seasoning for grilled chicken or fish. The possibilities are endless, so don't be afraid to get creative and try new ways to include spices and seasonings in your meals. Just be sure to choose low-sodium options and include them in moderation as part of a well-rounded and balanced diet.

Bonus Chapter
Flat Belly Recipes to Try

Here are a few flat belly recipes that you can try incorporating into your diet:

- ➢ Quinoa and Black Bean Salad:
  - 1 cup cooked quinoa
  - 1 cup cooked black beans
  - 1 cup diced tomatoes
  - 1 cup diced cucumbers
  - 1 cup diced bell peppers
  - 1/4 cup chopped cilantro
  - 2 tbsp olive oil
  - 2 tbsp lemon juice
  - 1 tsp cumin
  - Salt and pepper to taste

Put all the ingredients together in a big bowl and mix well. Serve chilled or at room temperature.

- ➢ Berry Smoothie Bowl:
- 1 cup of frozen berries (such as raspberries, blueberries, or strawberries)
- 1/2 cup Greek yogurt
- 1/2 cup unsweetened almond milk
- 1 tsp honey (optional)
- 1 tsp chia seeds
- 1 tsp chopped nuts (such as almonds or walnuts)

Blend berries, yogurt, and almond milk together until smooth. Pour into a bowl and top with chia seeds and nuts.

- ➢ Grilled Chicken and Avocado Salad:

- 4 oz grilled chicken breast

- 1 cup mixed greens

- 1/2 avocado, sliced

- 1/4 cup cherry tomatoes, halved

- 2 tbsp olive oil

- 1 tbsp lemon juice

- Salt and pepper to taste

Put all the ingredients together in a big bowl and mix t well. Serve chilled.

> Roasted Vegetable and Legume Bowl:

- 1 cup cooked quinoa

- 1 cup roasted vegetables (such as bell peppers, onions, and zucchini)

- 1 cup cooked legumes (such as black beans or chickpeas)

- 1/4 cup chopped cilantro

- 2 tbsp olive oil

- 2 tbsp lemon juice

- 1 tsp cumin

- Salt and pepper to taste

Put all the ingredients together in a big bowl and mix well. Serve chilled or at room temperature.

➤ Salmon and Veggie Skewers:

- 4 oz salmon fillet, cut into chunks

- 1 cup cherry tomatoes

- 1 cup diced bell peppers

- 1 cup diced onions

- 2 tbsp olive oil

- 1 tsp lemon juice

- Salt and pepper to taste

Thread salmon and vegetables onto skewers. Brush with lemon juice, and olive oil, then season with pepper and salt. Grill until the salmon is cooked and the veggies are tender.

- ➢ Chickpea and Spinach Curry:
- 1 cup cooked chickpeas
- 1 cup chopped spinach
- 1 cup diced tomatoes
- 1/2 cup coconut milk
- 1 tsp curry powder
- 1 tsp garam masala
- Salt and pepper to taste

Put all ingredients in a pot and boil. Cook until the spinach is tender and the chickpeas are heated through. Enjoy over cooked rice or quinoa.

- ➢ Lemon and Herb Grilled Chicken:
- 4 oz chicken breast
- 2 tbsp lemon juice
- 2 tbsp chopped herbs (such as basil, parsley, or cilantro)

- 2 tbsp olive oil

- Salt and pepper to taste

Combine lemon juice, herbs, olive oil, and salt and pepper in a small bowl. Brush the mixture over the chicken and grill until cooked through.

➢ Cucumber and Dill Yogurt Dip:

- 1 cup Greek yogurt

- 1/2 cup diced cucumber

- 2 tbsp chopped dill

- 1 tsp lemon juice

- Salt and pepper to taste

Combine all ingredients in a small bowl and mix very well to combine. Serve with veggies or entire grain crackers for dipping..

➢ Tofu and Vegetable Stir-Fry:

- 4 oz firm tofu, cubed

- 1 cup mixed vegetables (such as bell peppers, onions, and broccoli)

- 2 tbsp soy sauce

- 1 tsp sesame oil

- 1 tsp honey

- 1 tsp grated ginger

Heat a large pan over medium-high heat. Add tofu and bake until both sides turned browned. Add vegetables and heat until tender. In a small bowl, Put soy sauce, sesame oil and honey and ginger in a small bowl and mix well. Pour the sauce over the tofu and vegetables and toss to coat. Enjoy over cooked rice or quinoa.

➢ Black Bean and Quinoa Salad:
- 1 cup cooked quinoa

- 1 cup cooked black beans

- 1 cup diced bell peppers
- 1/2 cup diced red onions
- 1/4 cup chopped cilantro
- 2 tbsp olive oil
- 2 tbsp lime juice
- 1 tsp cumin
- Salt and pepper to taste

Put all the ingredients together in a big bowl and mix well. Serve chilled or at room temperature.

➢ Roasted Vegetable and Hummus Wrap:
- 1 whole grain wrap
- 1/4 cup hummus
- 1 cup roasted vegetables (such as bell peppers, onions, and zucchini)
- 1/4 cup chopped spinach

Spread hummus over the wrap and top with roasted vegetables and spinach. Roll all the wraps and cut them in half. Serve chilled.

Overall, there are many delicious and nutritious recipes that you can include in your flat belly diet. Just be sure to choose a variety of ingredients and include them as part of a well-rounded and balanced diet.

Conclusion

How to Incorporate These Flat Belly Foods into Your Diet

Incorporating flat belly foods into your diet is easy. You can try adding a serving of these foods to your meals or snacks, or using them as a base for dishes like salads or bowls. You can also try incorporating these foods into your cooking, such as using leafy greens as a base for smoothies or using berries as a topping for oatmeal. Just be sure to choose a variety of these foods and include them as part of a well-rounded and balanced diet.

Here are a few tips to help you incorporate these flat belly foods into your diet:

- Plan Ahead: Planning your meals and snacks in advance can help you make sure you're getting a variety of flat belly foods throughout the week. You can try prepping some of these foods in advance, such as chopping vegetables or cooking grains, to make it easier to include them in your meals.

- Be Creative: Don't be afraid to get creative and try new ways to incorporate these foods into your diet. You can try using them as a replacement for less healthy ingredients or experimenting with different recipes and flavor combinations.

- Don't Forget Portion Sizes: It's important to remember that even healthy foods can contribute to weight gain if you eat too much of them. Be mindful of portion sizes and aim to include these foods in moderation as part of a well-rounded and balanced diet.

- Keep It Simple: You don't have to prepare elaborate meals to include these foods in your diet. Try keeping it simple by pairing these foods with other healthy ingredients and seasoning with herbs and spices.

- Don't Be Afraid To Try New Things: Experimenting with different types of flat belly foods can help keep your meals interesting and prevent boredom. Don't be afraid to try new types of berries, nuts and seeds, or grains. You might discover some new favorites!

- Make It Convenient: It's easier to include these foods in your diet if they are convenient to eat. Try keeping some of these foods on hand as grab-and-go snacks, such as a bag of nuts or a container of yogurt. You can also try packing some of these foods in your lunch or taking them with you when you're on the go.

Overall, incorporating flat belly foods into your diet is all about finding what works for you. Don't be afraid to experiment and try new things, and remember to include these foods as part of a well-rounded and balanced diet. With a little bit of effort and planning, you can easily incorporate these foods into your daily routine and work towards a trimmer waistline.

Final Thoughts

Incorporating flat belly foods into your diet can be an effective way to support weight loss and achieve a trimmer waistline. These foods are typically low in calories and high in fiber, which can help keep you feeling full and satisfied. They are also often rich in nutrients that are important for overall health, such as vitamins, minerals, and antioxidants.

When incorporating flat belly foods into your diet, it's important to choose a variety of these foods and include them as part of a well-rounded and balanced diet. Don't be afraid to get creative and try new recipes and flavor combinations, and remember to pay attention to portion sizes. With a little bit of effort and planning, you can easily incorporate these foods into your daily routine and work towards a flat belly.